How to get started in running – A 10 step plan

By Mark Wigley

Contents

Disclaimer

Before starting any new exercise or diet regime it is advisable to get advice from your GP or Physician to ensure that your new endeavour is safe to begin. Explain to them what you intend to do and get their advice on how, if and when to start. Nothing in these pages is designed to replace professional advice from a medical professional, qualified running coach or a dietician. If their advice differs from mine, then on the balance of probabilities they are probably correct! The information below is what worked for me and is only guidance. It is my sincere hope that you find some or all the information contained in this book useful in starting, continuing and enjoying running.

Introduction

Running, where do I start. I got into running about 2 and a half years ago. Prior to that I had dabbled a little bit with the pastime, the odd 10k here and there and a couple of half marathons; all many years ago. Back then I could take it or leave it. This time however running has stuck and it has got properly under my skin (and my feet) and into my life. In fact, I am not ashamed to say that I love running! Anyone who knows me will know that I totally lack fast reflexes, balance and hand-eye co-ordination and I lose interest quickly in any activity that has complex rules, activities, loads of equipment or is very difficult and time consuming to get even a little bit good at. I tried cycling (equipment and balance), martial arts (complex rules and activities) and golf (everything on the above list). Running has been the one and only thing that I have found that I can do and be a bit good at as well! I have grown to love running for several reasons:

1. Anyone can start running. Virtually anyone who is relatively able-bodied can have a go at running, it really is an everyman's sport. You don't need any expensive memberships, subscriptions, clothing or equipment to get started. All you need is a little bit of willpower, a half decent pair of trainers (or just go barefoot!) and some tarmac or a path and you are off!
2. When you run you set off the release of happy chemicals in the brain, running is a great way to relieve stress and be with your own thoughts.
3. Everyone is rooting for you. Running is extremely egalitarian. When you participate in a race everyone is cheering you on, no matter who you are, who you represent or what your level of ability is. Everyone gets a medal for completing a race, you even get one for coming last! A medal for coming last! Awesome!
4. Running burns calories. If you are trying to lose weight, then run. Running burns so many calories. The last marathon I did burnt nearly 5000 calories. Running is also very good for your overall health.
5. Running is linear, pure and simple. Although you can get into the science of running which covers topics from nutrition right through to the type of shoes you 'should' wear, running is pure and can take you back to what it felt like to run as a child. A few twists and turns aside, running just simply involves travelling in a straight line putting one foot in front of the other, faster than walking.
6. Sense of achievement. Regardless of whether you have just completed your first mile or your first marathon there is a massive sense of achievement that no-one can take away from you.
7. Meeting great people. Running has a huge community attached to it, from parkrun to small running groups. Great people, full of encouragement.
8. Giving something back. Support from the running community to help you achieve your goals is great, what is even better is helping other people achieve theirs. Some will marvel at what you can do and will want to follow you and you will marvel at others and want to follow them.
9. Even if you have a bad run you can still revel in the hardship and use it build your mental toughness
10. You may even find that running helps you develop in other parts of your life too.

This book is not a book about breaking records or coming first in running (neither of which I have done, to date!) It is just a book about running. I am hoping that you can use this book and apply the steps in these pages to help you get started, continue, improve, achieve and learn to love running.

Step 1 – Getting started

"It's a dangerous business, Frodo, going out your door. You step onto the road, and if you don't keep your feet, there's no knowing where you might be swept off to." JRR Tolkien, Lord of The Rings

So, you have decided to start running. Well done. Decision is the first step but certainly not the last. Commit yourself to going for that first run. Things to accept early on. You will probably hate it. You think you won't look good. You may not feel good and you may even never want to run again after your first attempt. These feelings are normal. If you feel any of these after your first run, you are my friend, a human being! That's good news. Your body already has many evolutionary adaptations that make humans better at running than most of the rest of the animal kingdom. Your brain has just forgotten this. It will remember.

The next step is action. Get up and go and get some comfortable clothes on. Shorts, jogging bottoms, t-shirt, hoody or just anything that you feel comfortable in. Find a pair of trainers out. Put them on. Go to the front door and step outside. Take a deep breath, exhale and then start putting one foot in front of the other at a faster pace than you would normally walk at your fastest. Keep doing this until you feel out of breath. Stop. Turn your head and look back at how far you have run. Congratulations you did it! The hardest part is done. It gets easier after this (honestly!)

It is important not to let the momentum go at this stage. Set a reminder on your phone for a couple of days' time to go running again. Your goal on your second run should be to run a little further than your first and so on and so on. Try and run (if you can) 2 – 3 times a week, allowing some rest in between. The goal is to gradually increase your distance and work on your stamina. Keep at it! You will be surprised how far you are running after just a few weeks.

Your first weeks might look something like this:

Day	Week 1	Week 2	Week 3	Week 4
Monday		1.5 mile		3.7 miles
Tuesday	0.5 mile		3.2 miles	
Wednesday		2 miles		3.9 miles
Thursday	0.75 mile		3.3 miles	
Friday		2.5 miles		4.1 miles
Saturday	1 mile		3.5 miles	
Sunday		3 miles		4.6 miles

It is a good idea to measure the distance you are running each time you go out. If you have a sports watch such as Garmin or Fitbit these will record the mileages for you. Or, you can pre-measure a route and then make notes using pen and paper afterwards. Keeping a record of well you are doing will help shut up the internal voice that will be telling you it is not working and that you should stop. There are also many free smartphone apps out there such as Strava that allow you to measure, capture and analyse data about your running.

Evolution of the human runner

Research points to our ancestors being 'persistence hunters'; unable to outsprint prey like deer we would track them at a slower running pace keeping them in sight and on the move until they became exhausted and could be killed.

Our physical anatomy has undergone many thousands of generations of evolutionary change to adapt us perfectly to run. Below are just some of them:

We possess a special ligament in the back of our head that stops it from tipping forward along with a flat face and teeth set back further in our head than other creatures. This gives us a better centre of gravity when running.

We are bipedal and stand upright meaning that only 40% of our bodies are exposed to the midday sun compared with 70% for other mammals. This allows our body to stay cooler in the hot sun.

Our nervous system produces chemicals that act as natural painkillers allowing us to offset a lot of the pain of running until after a run has been completed.

Unlike a lot of other mammals, we can lose body heat through sweating as we have large numbers of sweat gland on our bodies and less body hair, this enables us to run for longer.

Humans also possess an extremely efficient breathing system which allows for increased airflow rates from lower muscular effort which also allows for a greater dumping of excess heat.

You see, you are a natural runner!

Step 2 - Dealing with Resistance and Setbacks.

"A setback is never a bad experience, just another one of life's lessons" Richard Branson

When you are starting any new endeavour that requires you to do something different you will have to deal at some point with resistance and setbacks. These tend to come from three sources, you, the people around you and the universe in general.

The Inner Voice (you).

Let's start with you. There is a little voice in your head that chatters away at you all day long, you may have probably heard from it already. For most people it acts as an internal critic and a safety adviser. These are some of the things your internal critic/safety adviser may say to you when you start running:

"That's too far"

"You can't do it"

"Give up"

"Don't go for a run" followed by "Why didn't you go for a run?"

"You can't breathe"

"Your legs hurt"

"You are not running fast enough"

"Everyone is better than you"

And so on and so on. Your inner critic/safety adviser only has one goal in mind when it chats away to you like this. TO STOP YOU FROM RUNNING. TO STOP YOU FROM CHANGING. TO KEEP YOU SAFE. Doing something different means changing, change means effort, effort brings risk of success, failure and uncertainty. Your inner voice will do all it can to put you off changing and then try and beat you up so bad afterwards you may never feel like changing again.

If you are going to keep moving forward, you will need to deal with this inner voice. I have discovered several ways you can deal with it.

1. IGNORE
2. RE-ASSURE
3. DEBATE

Out of all these methods I have found that the least successful method is to IGNORE the voice. The more you ignore it the more it tends to get louder and more insistent. If you can put up with this however, the tactic may work for you and buy you enough time to complete your run.

You can RE-ASSURE the inner voice with something like this:

Inner Voice: Legs are hurting, let's stop running.

You: Yes, they are hurting and thank you letting me know, now that I know that they are hurting I will monitor the situation and if necessary, stop and rest, how does that sound to you?

Inner Voice: Ok for now, but I will be coming back to this.

You: That's fine, I love you for caring.

What you are doing here is letting your brain know that you have recognised a potential problem and are prepared to deal with it if it becomes more serious. This may buy you enough time to carry on by placating your inner voice that everything is under control.

Another option is to DEBATE with your inner voice; as it is always right it will usually relish the opportunity to argue with you. This again may buy you enough time to complete your run. It might sound something like this:

Inner Voice: You won't be able to run 4 miles today.

You: Why do you say that I ran 3.7 miles only the other day.

Inner voice: Yes but its 4 miles, you were very tired the other day when you finished.

You: I was but look I am at 3.8 miles now we are almost there.

Inner Voice: It's still too far for you to run.

You: Oh, look I have just run 4 miles.

Notice I talked about buying yourself time with these tactics, the inner voice for most of us is undefeatable and always right. Because of this we can only do our best to bog the inner critic down long enough to get our shit done.

Other people.

Fortunately for most people who start a brave new endeavour they get ample support from friends, family and partners and I hope (like me) you fall into this category. However sometimes the people around you can often be resistant and even hostile to the changes that you are starting to make in your life, especially when they see those changes take you away from time with them. These types of behaviours usually come from love, fear, anxiety and even jealousy. They love you and don't want you to get hurt or fail, scared because you might succeed and leave them behind and anxious because they may not fully understand the need for change in your life. They may also become jealous as you are out there trying new things, meeting new people and having a blast without them needing to be there. It is important to recognise when this resistance is coming or is happening so you can have a strategy to deal with it. You could:

1. IGNORE
2. EXPLAIN
3. SIGN THEM UP
4. RECRUIT THEM

You could try and IGNORE the complaints and concerns from your family, friends and partner and just get on with it. This is a high-risk strategy as you may come across as un-caring and obsessed. It may however work if you just have to put them off for a very short period of time and you can always deal with the fallout afterwards.

The second option is to take some time to sit down with you partner, family and EXPLAIN to them your plan and why doing this is important to you and what you want to achieve from doing it. Hopefully they will understand and be ready to support you.

The third option is to SIGN UP your family members to running; if you can get them to join in with your running then it becomes a family endeavour which you can all enjoy together. You will be able to bring everyone along with you on the journey. It's a win-win.

Another option is to RECRUIT them as cheerleaders for your running adventures. If you can get your partner/family members to come along to your events and cheer you on, or get them involved with fundraising for you (if you decide to do a sponsored run) or even make a family weekend away to attend a race then you will have a better chance of avoiding hearing the following phrases (or similar) from your loved ones:

"You should be happy with what you have"

"Play it safe"

"You've changed"

Events

The other route through which you might get resistance and setbacks is from the "universe" or "life" or "the world" or however, you choose to describe the source of events that seemingly come out of nowhere and disrupt your plan.

These setbacks can include injury, cancelled runs, the weather, family tragedy, illness and many others. All these provide perfect opportunities for your Inner Voice to convince you to abandon your running plans entirely.

When these events occur take a deep breath, calm down and rationally assess the impact of the event on your running plans. It is very rare that the event will cause you to have to give up running permanently or even stop running at all. Consider:

1. What has happened?
2. Will it necessarily stop me running?
3. Will running help me get through the situation?
4. If it is going to stop me running, how long for?
5. When is the earliest I can get back to running and put a date in the diary to get re-started?

I have provided the following example below to illustrate how the 5-step plan could work for you if you face a setback.

John is a runner who has just found out that he has lost his job. He is stressed, anxious, angry and scared about the situation as he has bills to pay and a family to support. He is feeling the pressure of having to get another job. The last thing on his mind is going running. Let's apply the 5-step plan to John's situation.

1. What has happened, John has lost his job.
2. Will it necessarily stop him running? No, you don't need a job to be able to go for a run
3. Will running help John get through the situation? It may do, running is known to release brain chemicals that relieve stress so continuing to run might help John get through his tough time.
4. Is it going to stop John running? Possibly for a little while whilst he uses the extra time to look for another job.
5. When is the earliest John can back to running? Well, let's say that John estimates it will take him a month to get another job. If he is going to stop whilst job-hunting, he could set a date in his diary for one month's time to go running.

This system can be applied to even the gravest of situations, even something as awful as a bereavement in the family.

The purpose of this section is to show you that despite setbacks and resistance from different sources you can find your way through them and continue with your running.

On a final note, one way you can help yourself when it comes to your family and friends is not to become a 'running bore'. You may have fallen in love with running and want to talk about it incessantly however you will quickly find that other people may not understand or care what you are talking about and you as well as them will end up getting frustrated. Talk about other stuff that isn't running! It's tough, I can talk about running all day long! Running is awesome!

Making time, not finding time.

When starting any new endeavour in life like running you will need to MAKE time for it. This is different from FINDING the time. Setting aside specific blocks of time in your life for running rather than just going running when 'you have the time' to do so is the key here. We all lead crazy busy lives and unless we schedule time in our diaries for events then they will be unlikely to happen at all. We all only have 24 hours in a day; most of them taken up with working and sleeping. Some of the remaining hours are taken up with commitments like family, leaving a few hours for proper free time. Sadly, many people don't undertake additional self-development in their lives because they claim, "they don't have time". They haven't made time. Look at your current schedule and see what other activities you can cut back on to accommodate your running. Something else will have to be sacrificed. I recommend replacing some of your TV watching time or your lie-in time at the weekend (if you are lucky enough to get any). This is un-productive downtime and doesn't really add any value to your life. For example, I run in the evenings after I get home from work and early on Sunday mornings. For my long Sunday morning runs I am usually back home before most of my family is awake still giving me the whole day with them. Carve out time in your schedule and block it out for running and protect those time slots ferociously. Nothing short of the apocalypse should allow one of those slots to be missed. The key lesson from this that if running is set in your diary for a specific day, time and duration the rest of your life will usually organise itself around those slots. Plan your running a week in advance and let everyone know what you will be doing.

Step 3 – Join the community

"Alone, we can do so little; together, we can do so much" – Helen Keller

By now you will have built up some extra confidence and self-esteem and you should now start seeing some results from your efforts. Provided you have been getting out regularly enough and putting it in your stamina will be improving and with it the distance you are able to run. To put it bluntly you won't be feeling like a 'bag of shit' every time you go out for a run.

Once you feel you are ready you can start looking around to see what the running community is like in your area. Trying to improve your running on your own is self-sabotage, you are not a superhero (although you may be feeling like one right now!) so finding individuals and groups out there will help you massively. If you are on Facebook, then a quick search for running groups will turn up some results. Check out the group and if you like the look of it message the group and go along for a try out session. These groups are invaluable in bringing along your running. They cater for all abilities and are usually very supportive of newbies. They normally organise meets during the week and at weekends and often put on all sorts of different events. Best of all most of them are free! The organisers do it for the love of running, not for profit. You get help with your running from those better than you and you can help those that are not. Keep your ego in check, stay humble and be a good runner and you will gain loads.

Another part of the running community is the growing phenomenon of Parkrun. Parkrun organises weekly (always 0900 on a Saturday morning) free timed runs in parks all over the world including the UK and US. The distance is always 5km. You register online and print off a barcode which you take with you to the run. After you finish your barcode is scanned by the volunteers that staff the run and your position and time is logged on a website where you can access your information. One of the best things about parkrun is the portability of your barcode; you can take it to any parkrun and run it and get scanned and recorded for it! Great when you are away from home on a weekend. Take your running kit with you! The field of runners that turn up at parkrun include elite runners that whizz round in under 20 minutes and those that get around in an hour, and the total number can be in the hundreds! Parkrun is a great way to start your weekend.

Pacing yourself.

Learning to pace yourself will be an important skill to learn if you want to really improve as a runner. It is very tempting to dash off heroically at the start of a race when you are feeling motivated and full of energy only to find later in the race that your pace collapses because you have worn yourself out. The pace that you run at will be affected by many other factors as well such as terrain, elevation, temperature, humidity, the weather, wind direction, your mental state, physical condition and the effectiveness of your pre-run and mid-run hydration and nutrition strategy. For example, you may be able to fly along at an even 9-minute mile on relatively flat tarmacked roads and then find when you hit the trails your pace drops to 13-15-minute miles or even a brisk walk on steep uphill's. With the advent of fitness tracker apps and watches you can monitor in real time your average pace and make necessary adjustments as you go. Your pace will also be different based on the distance you are running and the goal you are looking at (are you shooting for a PB or is it just a relaxed social run) achieving. On something like a 5km run you will be looking at a much faster pace than you would go for if you were running a marathon. Work out different paces for different runs and then work on improving them.

Step 4 – Participate

"Winning has a value for ego, but participation has a value for life." — Debasish Mridha

Wow, you have come a long way by now, you may be running regularly on your own, with friends and family and/or with a running group. You may even have done a few parkruns (and even have claimed your first parkrun t-shirt!). Awesome.

Whilst out running with other people you will have surely heard other runners talking about races that they signed up for or have completed. Your head will probably be buzzing with all the different types of races being referred to and terminology used. Like all hobbies and sports there is a whole new language to learn.

Also get on the internet and start looking for organised running events in your area (or beyond if you fancy travelling!). According to a survey conducted in 2014 by Sports Marketing Surveys Inc (link to survey at end of book) there were 10.5 million runners in the UK with half of those participating in at least one competitive event every year; you can imagine the size of the number now in 2019! This means that there is a whole industry dedicated to providing running events to cater for the mass of runners that are eager to sign up! Races vary in distance and difficulty, can be on-road and off-road and keep going up to insane distances and difficulties. All are inexpensive to enter and start at single-digit amounts up to triple-digits depending on the type of race. All abilities from elite downwards enter these races with only a handful of races having qualifying requirements (usually the ones reserved for utter lunatics). Everyone who completes one of these races will get a medal and sometimes even a free t-shirt! You get a medal even if you come last! Talk to a few people about the races they have entered and ones they have completed and see if any of the events resonate with you. Once you have found one, sign up for it! The goal is not to pick something that is absolutely going to kill you, just one that you will be able to comfortably train for and complete, something to build your confidence. Once you have entered the race you can immediately start to train for it. A trick here is not to pick something so far off in the future that you will never start training for it and not something so close you will not have time to adequately train for it. A 10km race for example will probably require about 8-10 weeks training depending on your current level of fitness. Longer races such as half-marathons, marathons and ultra-marathons will take longer. In fact, a 10km race is a great place to start when entering your first race. It is relatively short and requires a small commitment of time for training so most runners can fit the training into their lifestyle. Train to finish the race in a time that is going to push you a little bit but not break you. Remember the goal is to finish, get your medal and then…. sign up for your next race! Provided you put it in adequately with the training, come race day you will be fine. Get to the venue in plenty of time to allow time for parking, registration, collecting race number, going to the toilet x 3 and wondering what on earth you are doing there. Nerves are normal, try and channel the nerves into energy for the race. Once the race begins get out there and have fun. You will get massive amounts of support and encouragement from other runners, spectators, marshals and even your own team of cheerleaders. There is nothing like the feeling of crossing that finish line and you will probably be somewhere in between bursting into tears and screaming with joy and collapsing on the floor and jumping with joy. Times and positions are usually published later the same day on the organiser's website, so you check how you did and where you came. You will normally be surprised to find that you didn't come last! Ok so now you have 24 -72 hours to bask in the glory of your achievement (and you deserve it) and then it's time to…. sign up for your next one.!

Developing mental toughness

I believe that about 50% of running is physical and 50% is mental. Look to push yourself to and sometimes beyond what you think you can do as much as you can and you will start to build the mental grit to be able to push your body further and harder even when your muscles and your inner voice is telling you to its time to stop. If you suffer a bad race and things do not work out well use that experience to your advantage and you will learn for next time and be able to overcome any problems if they occur again. Don't look at a bad race as a failure; look at it as a positive learning experience. Analyse what went wrong and think about what you might do differently next time. The great thing about developing the mental toughness in running is you will find it will make you more resilient in other areas of your life.

Step 5 – Set a stretch goal

"What you get by achieving your goals is not as important as what you become by achieving your goals." – Henry David Thoreau

Awesome, the last few months have been quite an adventure for you. You will have started to experience the highs and lows of being a runner. At this stage you may have already participated in 2 or 3 races and are starting to rack up a collection of t-shirts and running bling. You are running regularly with a group and can share stories of your runs with others. Share the bad times as well as the good times. No-one is a perfect runner, and everyone has a bad run occasionally, it's all part of the rich tapestry of being a runner. Don't moan too much about your bad runs and don't brag too much about your good runs, stay humble and try and listen more than you talk. If you listen well, you can pick some great advice about how to improve your running. Taking advice comes with the following caveats. There is an abundance of advice out there about running and it tends to fall into the following categories:

1. Scientifically proven
2. Useless and/or dangerous
3. Based solely on the personal experience of the adviser
4. Has some scientific research behind but needs more
5. Received wisdom (advice that is commonly held to be true, but might not be true)

My advice (which of course you don't have to follow) is to listen to all advice you are given, do your own research into it and follow the advice you think will work for you. Advice is advice, it's not mandatory! There are lots of opinions and studies on everything from hydration strategies through to the type of shoe you should wear. One trick I have learnt is that if you do hear someone giving advice that you think is nonsense NEVER try and correct them in front of other people. You will cast them and yourself in not a very good light which won't go down very well. Nobody likes having their ego bruised and nobody likes an ego-bruiser. It is other people's own responsibility to go off and check if what they have been told is true and I recommend you do this with the information in this book too! For the most part though you will pick up some wonderful little gems of advice that you can take away and apply to your own running.

Now it's time for the big one, setting a stretch goal. Find a quiet place away from all distractions (yes, put your phone away) and sit down. Close your eyes and relax, taking some slow deep breaths. Allow your mind to clear and whilst taking in those slow deep breaths ask yourself the following questions:

"What is the longest race I can imagine myself doing?"

"How many miles would it be?"

"How would I feel when I finish it?"

Try and visualise yourself running the race, feeling the ground underneath your feet, the feeling of exertion in your breathing and the elation of crossing the finishing line.

Once you have done this open your eyes, return to the room and write down that distance on a piece of paper. Now go to the internet and find a race that is slightly further than you can imagine running in one go. That is your stretch goal. That is the race you need to enter.

For example, Helen imagines running and has written down 10 miles as the distance. She goes onto the internet and finds a half marathon (13.1 miles). That's the race she enters.

The reason for picking something further than you think you can run is to start getting into the habit of pushing yourself beyond what you can comfortably do (known as your comfort zone). You can do more than you think, and you can go further than you can imagine. Make sure you follow the guidance about allowing just enough training time for your chosen run.

I chose my stretch goal in June 2018. I had completed a few races and was looking around for something to do in the late summer. I did the above exercise and could visualise myself completing a marathon (26.2 miles). I went online and looked for something slightly further than a marathon and found a 31-mile ultra-marathon. That was my stretch goal, out of my comfort zone and that was the race I needed to enter!

This is not a book about training programmes, there are loads to choose from out there on the internet and in books and publications on training plans. Find a training plan that suits your lifestyle and commitments and its game on!

Provided you put it in adequately with the training, come race day you will be fine. Get to the venue in plenty of time to allow time for parking, registration, collecting race number, going to the toilet x 3 and wondering what on earth you are doing there. Nerves are normal, try and channel the nerves into energy for the race. Once the race begins get out there and have fun. You will get massive amounts of support and encouragement from other runners, spectators, marshals and even your own team of cheerleaders. There is nothing like the feeling of crossing that finish line and you will probably be somewhere in between bursting into tears and screaming with joy and collapsing on the floor and jumping with joy. Times and positions are usually published later the same day on the organiser's website, so you check how you did and where you came. You will normally be surprised to find that you didn't come last!

Food and Drink

This is not a book about diet and nutrition, and I am no saint when it comes to eating right so this will be a very brief section. All I will say is that as soon as you start your running start thinking about what you are putting into your body. You will be developing into a new and improved souped-up version of your previous self and this new running machine will require better fuel to be put in the tank. Running is a good opportunity to look at and change where necessary bad eating habits and start eating right. You will need to think about what you eat when you are not running, before you run and whilst you are running and there is much advice out there on how to do this (way outside the scope of this book) including what to eat during a race. Hydration is important too. Drink more water. Again, there are articles on hydration strategies for race day as well. The only advice I would give you is to start paying more attention to the food you are putting into your body and try and steer clear of highly processed foods.

Step 6 – Rest

"There is virtue in work and there is virtue in rest. Use both and overlook neither" – Alan Cohen

Now that you have achieved your stretch goal you might find that you feel a little bit beat up so it's time for a period of recovery and rest. There is no exact formula for how long this period should last for however I saw an article in Runnersworld (link to article in references) that recommends 1 day of rest for each mile ran. So, if you have just completed a marathon then 26 days of rest and recovery are recommended. This does not mean a complete break from exercise altogether or even from running entirely and certainly not a return to the couch! Get out and enjoy some walking and/or other forms of exercise and gradually re-introduce some gentle running over the duration of the recovery period. Rest and recovery are both important in order to get you back into proper running form again. If you don't allow ample time to recover then you risk returning to running and carrying niggling little aches, pains and injuries around with you that will not only reduce your performance but also make you start to hate running. So, to conclude this section you can bask in the glory of your stretch goal achievement for 1 day per mile you ran! Rest and recover and get yourself ready for your return.

Warming up, warming down and stretching.

You may find it beneficial to do some form of warming up and warming down before and after a run, especially for strenuous and/or long runs. I favour dynamic stretching and a short warm up run before a run and then a short walk/slow run to warm down afterwards. When it comes to stretching there are different types of stretching like static and dynamic stretching. Most runners will do some form of warming up and warming down and there are those that do more than others. Do your own research into the benefits of stretching and you will probably find as many studies that suggest stretching works as you will suggesting that stretching doesn't work. Work out a routine that works for you.

Step 7 – Taking it to the next level

"Your strength doesn't come from winning. It comes from struggles and hardship. Everything that you go through prepares you for the next level." - Germany Kent

You are such a legend! In the last few months you have started an amazing new hobby which is great for your physical and mental wellbeing, stuck at and smashed your stretch goal. Now that all the hubbub has died down you may be asking yourself where you can go from here. You may have decided that achieving such a huge goal is enough or (as is very common with runners) you are looking for more.

It's time to take it to the next level and really start running to ramp up your performance and stamina. Start looking around for your nearest UK Athletics affiliated running club. These clubs cater for elite competitive runners and for those who are looking to drastically improve their running ability. Most offer a free try out session that you can go along to and most are low cost to join. You will need to become a member of UK athletics and this will also get you discounts on any races you enter after joining. Sessions are held during the week and at weekends and you will get the opportunity to represent your club at competitive races as well. Running with and being around runners that are significantly better than you is a sure-fire way of taking your running to the next level. You will come with some running history and some races under your belt so you will have enough credibility to fit in with the group. The rest is up to you. Push yourself hard at each session, listen to the advice and watch how others run and you will find that in a very short amount of time everything about your running will improve, endurance, speed and technique. I procrastinated for far too long about joining a running club but when I finally did, boy! Did my running take off! You bet it did. There is also something about wearing a vest with the name of your running club on it during a race, you almost feel obliged to run harder and do better as you are representing your club and your team are depending on you.

If you like the social aspect of club membership these running clubs have an active social calendar with events and awards ceremonies, so you not only get to run better you also get to party a little as well.

To wear or not to wear.

Choosing what to wear or not to wear when running is another part of the planning and preparation for running. Personal preference and practical considerations need to be balanced to make sure that you are going out on a run dressed for optimum performance. It's very tempting on a cold winters day to wrap up in a hat, gloves and thick clothing because you are cold only to find that a few miles into the run you are baking hot and overheating from exertion. A great bit of advice I heard is to start running in what you will most want to be finishing in. Running creates a lot of heat in the body so you will want to finish the race without being boiling hot. You can always put on warmer clothing after the race has finished, after you have cooled down. Remember that heat is a runner's enemy and if you overheat it can drastically reduce your performance!

Step 8 – Set a new stretch goal

"If you want to be happy, set a goal that commands your thoughts, liberates your energy and inspires your hopes." —Andrew Carnegie

In this step you can repeat the same visualisation process that you completed in Step 5 which I have repeated below for you for your convenience:

Find a quiet place away from all distractions (yes, put your phone away) and sit down. Close your eyes and relax, taking some slow deep breaths. Allow your mind to clear and whilst taking in those slow deep breaths ask yourself the following questions:

"What is the longest race I can imagine myself doing?"

"How many miles would it be?"

"How would I feel when I finish it?"

Try and visualise yourself running the race, feeling the ground underneath your feet, the feeling of exertion in your breathing and the elation of crossing the finishing line.

The distance you visualise should hopefully be further than the race you ran in your first ever stretch goal!

Once you have done this open your eyes, return to the room and write down that distance on a piece of paper. Now go to the internet and find a race that is slightly further than you can imagine running in one go. That is your second stretch goal. That is the race you need to enter.

For example, Helen has previously run a half marathon as her first stretch goal. She does the visualisation exercise again and imagines herself running and has written down 15 miles as the distance. She goes onto the internet and finds a marathon (26.2 miles). That's the race she enters.

I chose my second stretch goal in January 2019. I had already completed my first stretch goal which was the 50k ultramarathon race back in the Autumn of 2018 and had joined my local running club to improve my performance. After doing the visualisation process, I came up with a longer distance and then found a run further than that which turned out to be 100k ultra-marathon which I am training for at the time of writing.

Follow the same process for training and completing the race as detailed in Step 5.

Running form and technique.

Observe any mass of runners and you will notice that pretty much everyone has their own unique form and technique. Unless your running form is affecting your performance or causing you problems my advice would be not to worry about it too much. If are determined to change your form and technique start gradually and try and find someone (preferably a running coach) to teach you the perfect running form and give you feedback on how you are doing. If you try and change your technique overnight, you can run the risk of causing yourself an injury.

Step 9 – Stay humble.

"Humility is really important because it keeps you fresh and new" -Steven Tyler

Well done you are now a seasoned runner, you have loads of runs under your belt and a shelf full of medals and a drawer full of race t-shirts. You can feel proud of all the achievements and hopefully by now your family and partner will be looking at you a lot differently than they did when you first sat down and laid out your running plans to them back in Step 2.

Remember that first running group you joined? There is a good chance that your running endeavours and hard work have put you way ahead of the other members of the group and you may find yourself running with them less and less as you train for longer events and improve your performance. If you can do it try and keep running with that group; don't forget where you came from and all the support and encouragement they gave you when you were a newbie. To the less developed runners in the group you will start to gain legendary status and they will be so pleased at how much you have achieved. Now it is time to try and give something back to those people. Run alongside the slower paced runners offering encouragement and support to them. Go to their races and cheer them on as they cross the finish line; remember they will have probably been doing it for you when you were starting out. Tell your stories and share the good times and the bad times. It is easy to turn up and just streak off ahead showing how fast you are, but it does not display gratitude and love to your fellow runners who have been there to pick you up and cheer you on. Save your best training runs for other times or with your official running club. A nice supportive social run at a steady pace can really put a smile on your face and contribute to keeping you in love with running. Celebrate your achievements but stay humble and you will have a solid support network of running friends for years to come.

Race day – Agony and Ecstasy.

By the time race day comes you will be raring to go. It is time to reap the benefits of all the planning and hard work you have put in preparing and training for the big day. There are no guarantees that everything will go entirely to plan but you have done as much as you can to mitigate any problems that might occur. Make sure your preparation continues in the hours leading up to the race:

1. Decent meal the night before
2. A good night's sleep
3. Get up early enough so you can have a decent breakfast and some fluids.
4. Get to the race venue early enough to get parked and pick up your race number etc. You don't need the added stress of getting their late and having to rush everything.

Once the race starts RUN YOUR OWN RACE BASED ON YOUR INTENDED PACE AND ESTIMATED FINISH TIME. If the person running next to you hares off ahead of you at the start don't be tempted to try and keep up with them, they may have a completely different race strategy from you or no strategy at all. If you have planned for a 10-minute mile pace, then stick to it. If in doubt start slow you can always make a little time back later.

If you suffer a problem on the run, try and analyse it rationally and calmly and decide what you are going to do about it.

On longer runs if you get a small niggle early on try and deal with at as soon as possible, a small niggle on mile 3 can become a major problem later in the race.

Use the mental toughness that you have been developing over time to get yourself across the finish line!

Step 10 - Keep going.

"As long as you keep going, you'll keep getting better. And as you get better, you gain more confidence. That alone is success" – Tamara Taylor

Step 10 is to keep going with running for as long you enjoy doing it. There may come a time in your life when you feel like stopping forever, or just taking a break for a while. The great thing is that all the things you have achieved with your running goals will stay with you forever and be another part of your life's rich tapestry. I know and have seen many runners who are still running in their 50's 60's and even 70's so advancing age is not necessarily a reason to stop. I have set my stop point at the 'race that will physically and mentally break me'. Even though I have staggered, swayed, hobbled and cried myself over many finish lines I am yet to find the run that will put me off the hobby forever. My search continues, and I hope it does for you to! Happy running.

References.

https://www.sportsmarketingsurveysinc.com/uks-running-population-reaches-remarkable-10-5m-says-sports-marketing-surveys-inc/

https://www.rei.com/learn/expert-advice/how-to-pace-your-run.html

https://www.runnersworld.com/training/a20854966/when-should-i-return-to-training-after-a-marathon/

https://www.parkrun.org.uk/

About the Author.

Mark has been an avid runner since 2017 and has been a member of Colchester Harriers Athletic Club since 2019. He has taken part in parkruns, half-marathons, marathons and ultra-marathons. Mark lives in Essex with wife Helen (also a keen runner), 2 boys and a couple of crazy dogs. For work Mark runs his own first aid training company and online course provider.

You can follow his running exploits on Instagram by following mark.wigley

www.ingramcontent.com/pod-product-compliance
Lightning Source LLC
Chambersburg PA
CBHW020333290526
45785CB00007B/3043